The Patient's Guide

Mammography

ADAM E. M. ELTORAI
TISHA M. SINGER
TERRANCE T. HEALEY

Praeclarus Press, LLC
©2019 Tisha M. Singer. All rights reserved.

www.PraeclarusPress.com

Praeclarus Press, LLC
2504 Sweetgum Lane
Amarillo, Texas 79124 USA
806-367-9950
www.PraeclarusPress.com

DISCLAIMER
The information contained in this publication is advisory only and is not intended to replace sound clinical judgment or individualized patient care. The author disclaims all warranties, whether expressed or implied, including any warranty as the quality, accuracy, safety, or suitability of this information for any particular purpose.

ISBN: 978-1-946665-24-9
©2019 Tisha M. Singer. All rights reserved.
Email: tsinger@lifespan.org

Cover Design: Ken Tackett
Developmental Editing: Kathleen Kendall-Tackett
Copy Editing: Chris Tackett
Layout & Design: Nelly Murariu

CONTENTS

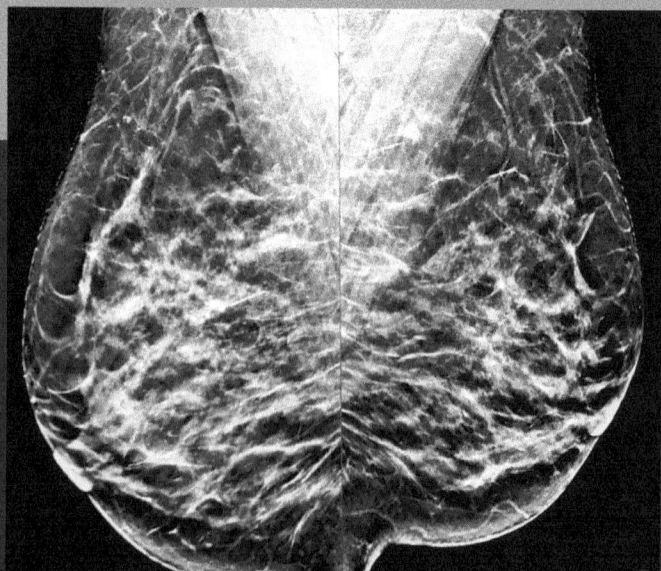

WHAT IS MAMMOGRAPHY?

Mammography is a type of radiology test where an X-ray picture is taken of your breast(s). It is most commonly used to check for the presence of breast cancer or to evaluate other issues that women may have, such as breast lumps or nipple discharge.

Screening Mammography

A screening mammogram is a type of mammogram that patients have when they have no signs or symptoms of cancer, or other breast problems. Women over the age of 40 come for a screening mammogram yearly. Many studies have shown that having yearly mammograms can help detect cancer at an earlier stage and prevent the number of deaths from breast cancer. Sometimes, women start having mammograms before the age of 40, most commonly due to a strong family history of breast cancer.

Diagnostic Mammography

A diagnostic mammogram differs from a screening mammogram and usually occurs to study an area of concern from a prior screening mammogram and/or to evaluate symptoms a patient is currently having, such as breast pain, nipple discharge, or a breast lump. Diagnostic mammograms are also done in women who are coming for 6-month follow-up exams for previously identified abnormal findings, for women with breast implants, and for women with a history of breast cancer.

Diagnostic mammograms are just like screening mammograms in that they are an X-ray picture of the breast, but instead of having a radiologist read the mammogram at a later time, this mammogram is read while the patient is still in the office. The radiologist may ask for more pictures of the breast, commonly known as spot or magnification views, to carefully study the area of concern. Patients may end up having more testing after diagnostic mammography, including tests such as breast ultrasound. Breast ultrasound is a different type of imaging which uses sound waves to show pictures of the breast and can often show different kinds of detail in the breast to help the radiologist better determine if an abnormal finding is benign or if it needs further evaluation.

THREE BASIC OUTCOMES FROM A DIAGNOSTIC MAMMOGRAM

1

The abnormal area on screening mammogram is found to be normal on additional views. When this happens, women can return to routine yearly screening mammograms.

2

The abnormal area on screening mammogram is not thought to be a cancer but the radiologist may want to follow this area closely. When this happens, women will return in 6 months for a diagnostic mammogram and/or ultrasound.

3

The radiologist thinks that the area of concern may or may not be cancer and will recommend that women undergo a biopsy of that area.

How Do I Prepare?

If you have a choice of where to go for your mammogram, try to choose a dedicated breast center that does many mammograms per day. If you do not know of a dedicated breast center in your area, ask your primary care provider or OB/GYN for a referral.

Ask the breast center you are considering going to if they do breast tomosynthesis. Breast tomosynthesis is a way of acquiring pictures of the breast that gives the radiologist many more views of the breast tissue at different angles. Breast tomosynthesis has been found to detect more early and subtle cancers.

If possible, always try to go to the same breast imaging center so they can compare your current mammogram with mammograms you have had in the past.

If you are going to a new facility for a mammogram, bring a list of other facilities where you had previous mammograms and/or breast procedures. If possible, bring any records of prior mammograms with you.

Choose the correct time of month to have a mammogram. Avoid going the week before your menstrual period and the first 5 days or so of your menstrual period. Try to pick a time of month when your breasts will not be tender.

Do not wear deodorant, powder, or perfume on the day of your mammogram. Deodorant and powder can create spots on the X-ray images. You can apply deodorant directly after your mammogram.

Dress appropriately and comfortably for your mammogram. Try to avoid wearing dresses and try to wear a two-piece item of clothing so that you can keep the bottom half of your clothing on during the examination.

Make sure to tell the mammogram tech that day if you think you could be pregnant.

Make sure to tell the mammogram tech that day if you are experiencing any problems with your breast, including any lumps, pain, or nipple discharge.

Ask when your mammogram results will be available, so you can make sure to call your primary care physician to follow-up with results.

QUICK LIST

✔ Try to choose a dedicated breast center.

✔ Ask for breast tomosynthesis.

✔ Try to go to the same breast imaging center.

✔ Bring a list of other facilities where you had previous mammograms and/or breast procedures.

✔ Have your records with you.

✔ Avoid going the week before your menstrual period and the first 5 days or so of your menstrual period.

✔ Do not wear deodorant, powder, or perfume on the day of your mammogram.

✔ Dress appropriately and comfortably.

✔ Inform the mammogram tech if you think you could be pregnant.

✔ Tell the mammogram tech that day if you are experiencing any problems with your breast, including any lumps, pain, or nipple discharge.

✔ Ask when your mammogram results will be available.

✔ Call your primary care physician to follow-up with results.

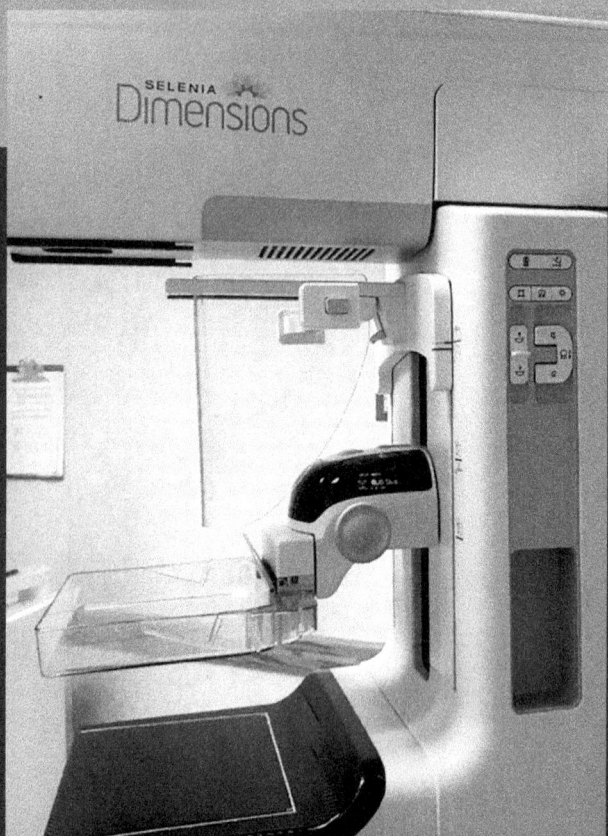

THE EQUIPMENT

A mammography machine is a rectangular shaped box that houses X-ray equipment used to take pictures of your breast. Mammography machines are used to take pictures of **breasts only** and cannot be used for X-rays of other body parts. There is a plastic device on the machine that is used to compress your breast so that better pictures can be taken.

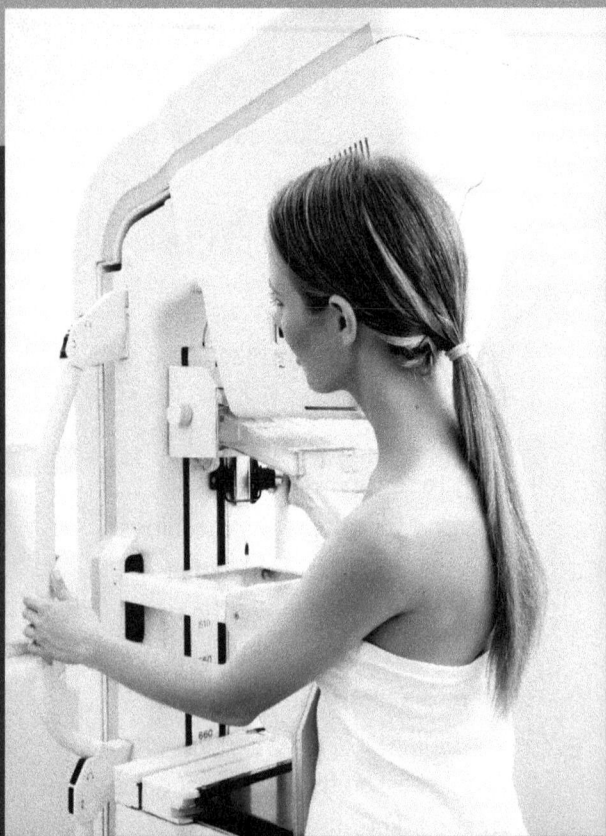

THE PROCEDURE PROCESS

Mammograms are performed on an outpatient basis. You will be asked to remove your top and/or remove the robe provided for the procedure so that your breasts are exposed.

The mammography technician will give you special directions to help position your breast on the mammography unit. A clear plastic paddle is used to compress your breast.

Many patients ask why we compress their breasts for mammography. Compressing your breasts helps us to see all of the breast tissue better and prevents breast tissue from overlapping. Other benefits of breast compression include lower radiation dose to the patient and clearer pictures for the radiologist to interpret.

After each picture is taken, the mammography technician will help to reposition your breast so that pictures can be taken from different angles. When pictures are being taken, you will be asked to stay very still and may be asked to hold your breath for a few seconds.

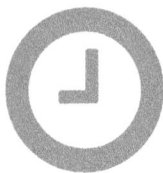

Usually the mammography tech will go behind a clear shield or will leave the room while the pictures are being taken.

The entire exam takes approximately 15-30 minutes from start to finish.

What Will It Feel Like?

You will feel pressure as your breasts are being compressed. This pressure may feel uncomfortable, especially if you have sensitive breasts. If you are feeling pressure that is too uncomfortable to tolerate, you can tell the mammography technician and they can lessen the amount of compression.

There are no needles or injections involved with mammography.

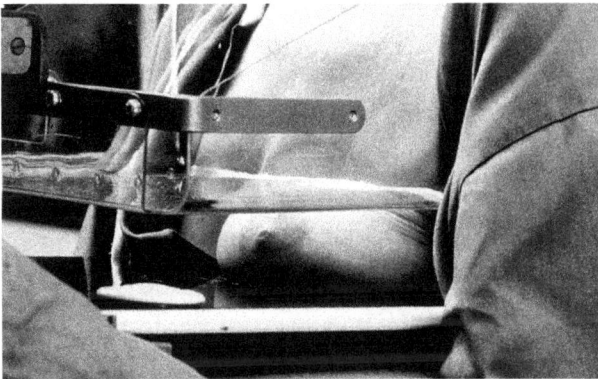

After the Procedure

If you are undergoing a screening mammogram, you can go home directly after the pictures have been taken. You will be notified in the next week or two if there is an abnormal finding on your mammogram. If your mammogram is normal, you will receive a letter in the mail notifying you of the normal mammogram within 30 days.

If you are undergoing a diagnostic mammogram, you will be asked to wait until the radiologist views the images. The radiologist may request that more X-ray images be taken, or may request an ultrasound as well. Before the end of your visit, you will find out the results of the mammogram and will be given direction if any further tests or imaging need to be done.

Results

As mentioned in the "after the procedure" section, a radiologist will view and interpret your breast mammogram.

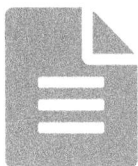

A radiologist is a physician trained to view and interpret X-ray pictures.

The radiologist will write a report about your mammogram and will send the report to your referring physician.

Just because you are called back for additional imaging, DOES NOT mean that you have a cancer.

Your referring physician will discuss the results of the examination with you.

If your mammogram is abnormal, the breast imaging center will contact you to make a follow-up appointment to come back for additional imaging.

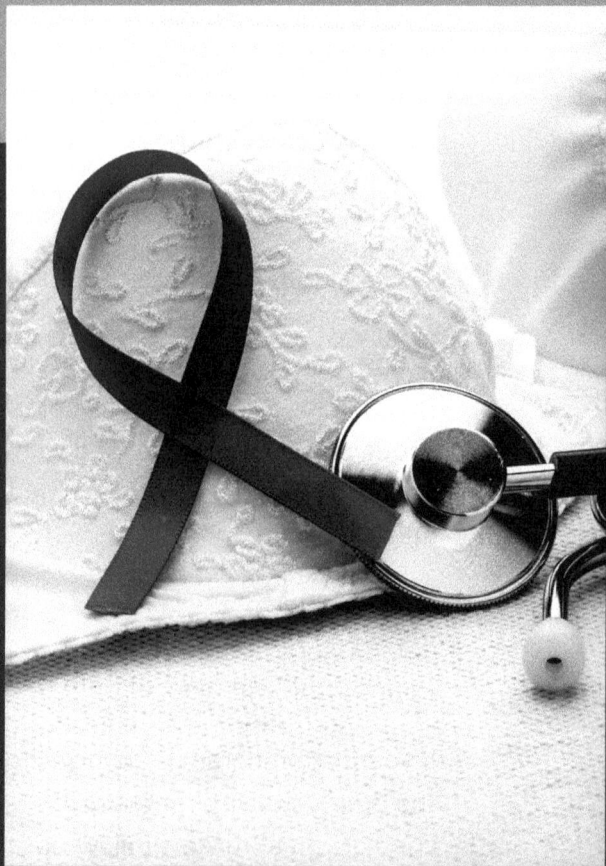

BENEFITS VS. RISKS

BENEFITS

Regular screening mammograms help to detect early breast cancer, possibly before the cancer has spread to other parts of the body.

Results from randomized clinical trials and other studies show that screening mammography can help reduce the number of deaths from breast cancer among women between the ages of 40 to 74, especially for women over the age of 50.

RISKS

Patients are exposed to a small amount of radiation from mammograms, although less than a standard chest X-ray.

Screening mammograms can be falsely positive and lead to additional imaging, which may cause worry, stress, and anxiety for patients.

LIMITATIONS

Mammograms do not detect every single cancer and may miss more subtle cancers.

Mammograms do not prevent women from dying from breast cancer. Some aggressive cancers progress quickly and can show up on mammogram when the cancer has already spread to other parts of the body.

FREQUENTLY ASKED QUESTIONS

How much does it cost to get a mammogram?

Most insurance plans cover screening mammography as a preventive benefit every 1-2 years for women age 40 and over without copayment. Many states require that Medicaid, Medicare, and public employee health plans cover screening mammograms.

If you do not have any form of health insurance, a mammogram costs between $80-$120.

There are many resources to help people who do not have insurance.

What kind of resources are available to help me pay for my mammogram? I don't have insurance.

For women who meet low income requirements, mammograms are covered by the National Breast and Cervical Cancer Early Detection Program. For more information, contact your state Department of Health.

Information about free or low-cost mammography screening programs is also available from NCI's Cancer Information Service at:

NCI's Cancer Information Service at 1–800–4–CANCER (1–800–422–6237)

If either of these resources are unavailable, you can contact your local hospital, health department, or women's health center to inquire about free or low-cost mammograms.

Do women over 40 with breast implants need screening mammograms?

Women with breast implants should undergo regular yearly screening.

There are special mammographic views which help to take pictures of your breasts without the implants in the field of view.

Make sure to tell the mammography technician that you have breast implants before the examination begins.

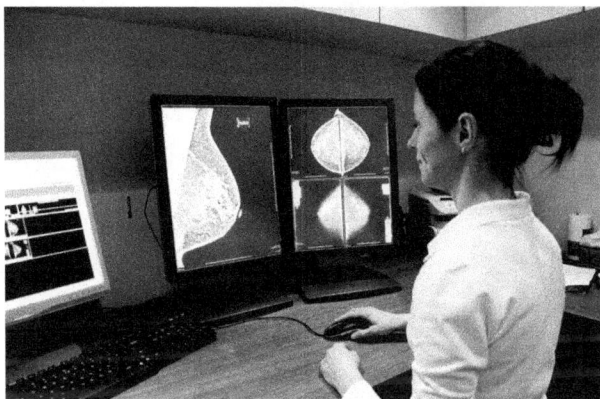

GLOSSARY

COMPRESSION

The process of compressing; the process of pushing or flattening by using light to moderate pressure

MAMMOGRAPHY

A technique using low energy X-rays to examine the human breast for both screening and diagnosis.

MAMMOGRAPHY TECHNICIAN

A person trained to operate radiology equipment that is used to take pictures of the breast to examine the breast for cancer and/or other abnormalities.

RADIOLOGIST

A medical doctor that specializes in treating and diagnosing diseases and injuries using medical imaging, such as X-ray, ultrasound, computed tomography (CT), positron emission tomography (PET), and magnetic resonance imaging (MRI).

ULTRASOUND

A type of imaging that uses high energy sound waves to form pictures of body parts.

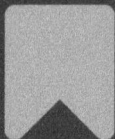

ADDITIONAL RESOURCES

cancer.org

cdc.gov

medlineplus.gov

KEYWORDS

● Mammogram ●

● Radiologist ●

● Breast cancer ●

MY CONTACTS

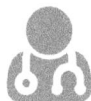

NAME	
CONTACT	

NAME	
CONTACT	

NAME	
CONTACT	

NAME	
CONTACT	

MY APPOINTMENTS

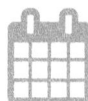

MONDAY

Date:
_____

THURSDAY

Date:
_____

TUESDAY

Date:
_____

FRIDAY

Date:
_____

WEDNESDAY

Date:
_____

SATURDAY

Date:
_____

MY QUESTIONS

MY QUESTIONS

MY NOTES

MY NOTES